I0411922

Running to a New Beginning

My Brain Rewired

By: John Canada III

[978-1507833797]

TABLE OF CONTENTS

Publishers Notes

Disclaimer

This publication is intended to provide helpful and informative material. It is not intended to diagnose, treat, cure, or prevent any health problem or condition, nor is intended to replace the advice of a physician. No action should be taken solely on the contents of this book. Always consult your physician or qualified health-care professional on any matters regarding your health and before adopting any suggestions in this book or drawing inferences from it.

The author and publisher specifically disclaim all responsibility for any liability, loss or risk, personal or otherwise, which is incurred as a consequence, directly or indirectly, from the use or application of any contents of this book.

Any and all product names referenced within this book are the trademarks of their respective owners. None of these owners have sponsored, authorized, endorsed, or approved this book.

Always read all information provided by the manufacturers' product labels before using their products. The author and publisher are not responsible for claims made by manufacturers.

Paperback Edition

Manufactured in the United States of America

Well, here I am seven months from my first marathon at forty seven years old. Had you said to me, "you will be running long distance for fun, fitness and sport", I would have thought you are crazy and said, "me"?

Forward

Epilepsy is a life-changing chronic disease. The "Running to a New Beginning" book described by Mr. Canada represents a collaborative process of destructive creation involving the epileptic patient at its center. Mr. Canada's epilepsy was interfering with his job, his daily activities with his family. Seizures could not be adequately controlled with medications alone. His desire to remain a helpful member of the society and lead a fulfilling family life, led him to continue to search for answers and best care, landing him at a level IV epilepsy center. It took a team work involving neurologist, neuropsychologist, radiologist, and neurosurgeon to conduct tests and identify the culprit portion of the brain causing seizures, the "epileptic focus".

The battery of tests also included functional tests to determine that it could be safely removed. The surgical resection was enhanced with intra-operative electrical recordings to insure safe removal of an adequate amount of tissue. Removal of brain tissue in this situation is certainly a destructive action; but, it allows the patients an opportunity to recreate the type of lifestyle they would like, given proper family and community support.

Mr. Canada was always engaged in the treatment process, understanding the risks of a major brain surgery while remaining optimistic. After a successful post-operative course allowed him to redefine himself with weight reduction, improved fitness, competitive running, and enhanced social interactions. His continued optimistic spirit and sense of community help has led him write this book and become involved with epilepsy foundation to provide for those who are looking for some hope in living with Epilepsy.

Dr. Rajdeep Singh

Epileptologist

Dr. Michael Heafner

Board Certified Neurosurgeon

Preface

After the last three years of my life, the accomplishments and trials I had faced, I felt compelled to write about epilepsy, running and me. I really would like to help others who may face adversity of any kind that it can be overcome. I was able to go back in time and remember how I felt growing up with epilepsy. I am excited to finally get my feelings of my life down on paper and expose how epilepsy had a profound effect on my life. I was surprised how some of the events in my life shaped my personality, beliefs and outlook on life.

As a first time author, I feel liberated writing about the story of this part of my life. I came to realize how important my life events were to others as they were to me. I was not ever one who intentionally looked to effect the life of others in a look at me sort of way. I just wanted to fit in.

Looking back I learned that what I thought about myself and "why was this happening to me" outlook was getting me nowhere. I found that a lot of great things happened in my life that I had all but dismissed. I now have a whole new approach to what's happening in my life now and what may come. There can be a joy amongst the trials knowing what has and will occur will be better than I ever thought.

I was surprised that once I started writing I didn't want to stop. I became dedicated to recalling the painful and joyous times in my life. I learned so much about epilepsy that I never knew before and was pleasantly surprised about things I was wrong about. The facts explained and reveal much about the events I experienced. It was refreshing that learning about being wrong was a great thing.

I asked people in my life to help me recall as much of the details of my life that I could. I cannot thank enough, my wife, Kristine, my daughters Meghan and Brianna, my parents, my brother and sister and my great friend Dan. Without them I couldn't have been the person I was and am today.

My doctors and medical staff were great in shaping my health into what it is today, Doctors, Rajdeep Singh, Johnnie Waataja and Michael

Heather to name a few. The staff of North Carolina Health Care System especially the Epilepsy Unit doctors and nurses were all fabulous.

Endorsement

In his book, John Canada takes us on his journey of coping with epilepsy from childhood through adulthood and his experience with uncontrolled seizures to life-changing surgery. He portrays the amazing resiliency of the human spirit in adapting to the burden of a chronic medical condition. Unlike many folks, he learns from his mistakes and has the good sense to make changes when needed. He is focused and driven to accomplish his personal goals. You find yourself rooting for him—run, John, run. You are an inspiration!

Patricia A. Gibson, MSSW DHL ACSW

Executive Director, Epilepsy Foundation of North Carolina

Dedication

I dedicate this book to my wife and daughters for continuing to push me forward.

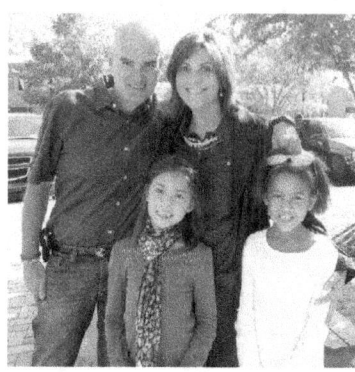

Chapter 1-

MY LIFE WITH EPILEPSY

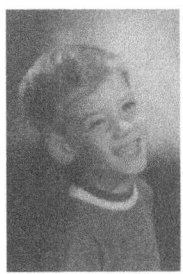

WHY AM I DIFFERENT

Epilepsy? What is that? Well for me it started about age five. I was getting notes to bring home for my parents. The letters spoke of how I was daydreaming in class. Unbeknownst to everyone, I was having seizures in school.

No one really understood what was happening, especially not me. Then, I had the first major seizure that I can recall. I was playing outside in the next door neighbor's yard, and then it happened. I fell to the ground without warning and started rolling around from side to side. I was really scared, because I was quite alert about what my body was doing but couldn't stop it.

Then the seizure ended just as quickly as it started. I remember lying down in the back seat of a car with my parents up front. I can only guess on the way to the doctor to find out why the seizure occurred.

ALL THE ACRONYMS

The first step was the barrages of tests need to find out why. The EEG (Electroencephalogram) which measures and records electrical activity in the brain, SPECT (Single Photon Emission Computed Tomography) which is a nuclear test that shows how blood flows to the organs and tissues, MRI (magnetic resonance imaging) which is used to take pictures inside the body, PET (Positron emission tomography) which is used to make three dimensional images of functional process in the human body. All of these and many others became a regular cycle.

For me the most frequent of this list was the EEG. I remember being told by the neurologist office that needed to stay up late the night before the test.

I thought great a valid excusable reason to stay up late. It was after the first few I realized I needed to be able to sleep during the test.

FLAT ON MY BACK

I arrived at the doctor's office each time and changed into a hospital gown. The next twenty minutes was spent rubbing my head in strategic spots along certain measurements of my skull. Then the cables were added. Each cable was placed to specifically track signals of the brain. After I was hooked up, I was told by the medical staff, " relax take a short nap". "Why?" I would ask. The quick reply, "We need you to be still so the test can give an accurate reading of your brain impulses". On one occasion I recall the medical staff telling me not to clench my jaw. I must have been doing it unintentionally. I thought I was sleeping well during the test after being up late but I heard the staff talking to me. There were so many images taken of my brain from age five until now. You would think I was being studied for how amazingly rare my brain was.

THE DIAGNOSIS

On a referral, the doctors sent my parents and me to the neurology center at the University of Miami in Florida. I was finally diagnosed with EPILEPSY. What is that?

Epilepsy is described as neurological disorder. The seizures are the product of the brain response to disturbing activity. There are a number of "generalized" seizures:

1)Grand-Mal myoclonic, tonic, clonic which causes uncontrollable body movements and unconsciousness and are the most violent and most likely to cause physical injury.

2)Absence seizures are described as a short loss of consciousness. The "partial" seizures include:

a) Simple partial that shows symptoms of rigidity, muscle jerking head turning, sensory disturbances to touch, taste, smell and vision.

b) Complex partial shows symptoms of lip smacking, chewing, fidgeting and repetitive involuntary movements.

I was definitely having complex partial seizures.

The symptoms I was having were consistent. So now that there was an actual diagnosis, the roller coaster of medication changes, constant blood tests, and regular office visits had become normal for my family and I.

BALANCING ACT

So now we have images of my brain. So what? The real work began. I was started on a regular dose of medication. The first medicine I recall was Phenobarbital. It was cherry flavor. I was good with that. I didn't really taste like medicine. That worked for a while and then it didn't. The balancing had started. I was then moved to a pill called Dilantin. That one was even better. It tasted like candy. So taking medicine wasn't so bad.

THE NEEDLE

The part of the balancing I wasn't particularly a fan of was the blood tests. After I gave so many vials of blood and after all this testing, the doctors were still not sure what was happening with me. The blood tests were definitely the most painful part of discovering what the right combination of medicines was going to be. My first couple of times I was getting stuck with a needle was as you would expect, unpleasant at best. The frequency of testing blood levels to tell if the amount of medicine in my system was sufficient enough to control the seizures varied as the weeks and months past. I became used to the needle in my veins located in the inside of the arm between the upper and forearm. It surprised me that there always seem to be one vein that would just "stand up" for the oncoming needle. It would say, "Another blood test? Not a big deal. Bring it on."

HERE THEY COME

I can tell you that for me it was the after affects of the seizures that were the only indicator to me that a seizure had even occurred. Each one, though a little different than the other, felt like there were pins and needles pricking me from the shoulders up to the top of my head.

The seizures themselves were not painful. It was being tired and the headaches that were the worst. It was so draining; I could lie down and sleep for hours on end. It was like all the energy was sucked out of my body through my skull. It really didn't matter where the seizure occured, I would be able to find a place to sit or lay down.

For everyone else on the other hand, it was upsetting to see and their question of why is this happening again always occurred.

When I was younger my family and close friends knew the seizures were occurring before I did. I denied the incidents happened to my family and I was aware that they knew better.

THE DENIAL

It was always denial for me about my seizures. It was my way of saying this is not going to stop me. I wanted control of my body and really new I didn't have any control.

The seizures caused an electrical storm in my brain. It was nothing like you would think. My seizures were quite silent. You wouldn't notice if weren't around me very often. The big cue for everyone was my body's lack of control of my attention span, awareness and muscle movements.

When out in public, if the episodes could be explained away they were. Sometimes my bladder control was affected too. My wet pants were often blamed on a ceiling or air conditioning leak or even a spilled drink. Anything to divert any "lookee loos" from asking any questions was the goal. Explaining away the seizures were quite aggravating for me. I didn't know the episode happened until after the episode was over.

It bothered me that I didn't know what happened and what people had seen. I was embarrassed until it was being questioned by people I didn't know. The same questions were "Are you okay?" "What happened here?" I was always wanting to say, "Everything ok, move on, nothing to see here!"Always being on the defense was tiring.

CLUES

There was always the question of how and why was this happening to me. Growing up, I was always so curious about it. I even researched epilepsy to find out what the causes must be. My initial findings were that the seizures were caused by a sharp blow to the head. I started to think if there were any times that I hit my head hard. Maybe it was the time I climbed out of the crib and fell on my head, breaking my collar bone. I wanted out of the crib and when crying to get out didn't work, I climbed out on my own at the highest part, the end of the crib.

OUTCAST

Going to school was particularly difficult for me even though I was going to a Catholic school. Making friends was hard, I believe, because I was so worried about other peers finding out about my seizures. I tried my best to keep seizures from anyone who didn't already know. It seemed that I was always being teased and ridiculed. I know some of the other students knew my secret. I tried to fit in to no avail.

I remember an incident in fourth grade when I had brought some comic books to share with the other students. I was made fun of again that day. My fourth grade teacher had enough of the other student picking on me. The whole class was taken to the side away from me and spoken to by the teacher. I didn't know what she said to them, but when they returned they were all so nice to me that day. It seemed that I was always going to be picked on so I just dealt with it. As you could imagine my self esteem was not great. I coped better as I advanced to each grade, partially because I mostly kept to myself.

FIRST CRUSH

There was this one girl I was quite smitten over during my last years in Catholic School, she was so pretty and popular. I tried to get to know her and even did a practice dance with her during one of our music classes to learn how dance. You know, hands on her waist, her arm on my shoulder with the formal personal space form. That was a great moment for me.

This girl was so heavily influenced by her friends that I never had a chance. Her friends that knew about my epilepsy were quick to talk her out of being my friend. Passing notes to her and trying to talk to her away from her friends didn't work. She was the first girl I really liked. So as you can imagine it broke my heart.

Chapter 2-

THE TEENAGE YEARS

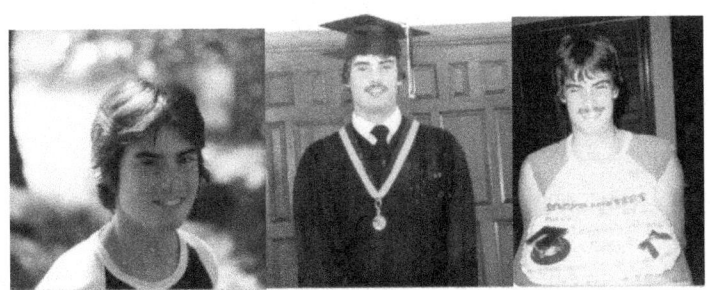

HIGH SCHOOL

When I entered Western High School, I was relieved that I didn't know any students. I was so introverted at that point that even approaching a girl was not a good experience.

I was still in a place of self loathing and pressure I put on myself to fit in. The possible connection to women at that time was few and far between. Don't get me wrong, most of the female contact I had was strictly due to classes, school related projects and sometimes lunch.

The girls I met during my first two years were more like acquaintances than solid friends. I usually only saw them at school. I had just given up on the concept of having a girl friend.

It wasn't until my junior year that a girlfriend became possible. Interestingly the girls I dated I met at events outside of school. Relationships were starting to be a great experience despite the epilepsy. My girlfriend from then on didn't even care about it. They liked me for me!

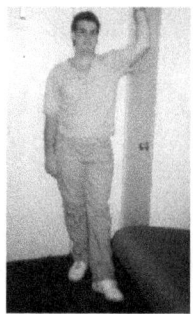

REAL FRIENDS

As far as high school friends and acquaintances go, my closer friends were really quite good about respecting me. I mean, like it or not, some of my friends were doing recreational drugs like marijuana and when they asked me to join them to smoke I said no.

I had a great shield in my epilepsy. I was able to use my medication and the fear of bad reactions to my meds and smoking or taking drugs as my excuse for not being able to participate.

It was quite good that despite my epilepsy I was not excluded or shunned from being friends with them. I was still able to hang out and have some understanding friends despite our individual vices. There was no judging from them or me.

MY BEST FRIEND

One day on the school bus during my sophomore year, I met Dan. We became fast friends after realizing that we both had the same favorite comedian, Bill Cosby. I was going through a few of the tracks from one of his albums. On the bus that day, I heard someone behind me reciting the same track. I turned around and met Dan, come to find out that we had so much in common. We both had Bill Cosby albums.

We started trading each other's albums and hanging out in school. We were such good friends even today, thirty-two years later. He was the outgoing one of the duo. He was there through all my ups and downs.

He tried on a few occasions, to get a girl or two to talk to me. It was great to have a friend that was really my friend, despite the epilepsy.

PASSIONS?

As far as a talent of mine, drawing was great way for me to express how I fit in to the world. I found drafting class was a class I enjoyed. My ability to draw floor plans and basic spatial drawing was great. I actually joined a public speaking club. We won a few debating matches which was great since I wasn't comfortable speaking to an audience. By then I felt that had better control of my seizures, since I was on a medication regiment that seemed to be working.

A SPORTING CHANCE

I also found some sports I liked. I tried out and got on the junior football team. My mom was resistant when I tried out because of my epilepsy. My dad convinced her to let me try. I was going to practice and doing well.

I was put in the position of right guard. Then one day at practice I went to block an opposing player and was easily knocked to the ground. I didn't remember getting hit. The coach was really concerned about the block and questioned what had happened.

I had become over heated and that brought on a seizure during practice that day. That ended football. I was on the hunt for a sport that I could enjoy. I found a bowling group that I could join with students from another high school.

I made a lot of friends through the high school bowling league. That became my sport of choice. It wasn't a contact sport and I was good at it. I was in more than one league at one point. I was bowling twice a week.

I was starting to feel more comfortable with myself and being around others. I wasn't worried so much about seizures being a focal point. I made some friends who knew about my seizures and it didn't matter!

SUPPORTING THE CAUSE

My epilepsy actually was great to have when I volunteered for a track and field Special Olympics event. I was paired with another athlete who happened to have epilepsy too. I was able to identify Buddy's seizures, support his running goals and be compassionate as well. Buddy had a seizure that day.

Another volunteer and I were able to get him off of the field so he wouldn't get hurt on the track. He had grand mal seizures. Contact with the ground there would have kept him from continuing the racing.

I actually felt like I knew what to do. I was able to keep him calm during his seizure and encourage him to resume his place in the games as an athlete. I felt like I was a part of Buddy's goals. I thought, maybe I might be able to be an athlete too.

It was great to be able to help someone who had a passion for track and field events. It is interesting how events come around and later return back into your life unexpectedly. I look back and wonder, should I have tried running back in high school?

Since that day Special Olympics has held a place in my heart. I can actually relate to what some of the athletes are going through. It is easier to understand the challenges they go through and how they still have such a positive and upbeat attitude and the desire to push past their physical limitations and play on.

BUILDING NEW CONNECTIONS

I was getting more confident about myself and my capabilities despite the epilepsy. I had continued my education in the area of Architecture at the local community college. I expanded my love of drawing, design and the styles of architecture throughout the world. I couldn't get enough of all aspects of creating and drawing buildings. I was particularly interested in Greek and Roman style of building and how they influenced each other. I became so passionate that some of my vacation spots were going to be Greece and Rome. I had done studies on

Egyptian pyramids, the pharaohs and their influence on architecture in the Middle East. I even got involved with the students in my design groups and the Architecture International Association (AIA). I got involved with a college fraternity that was very active in the Broward College social life. We were the support for all the social activities on and off campuses.

COLLEGE LIFE

My first taste of being initiated was at our first member's only retreat in Lake Placid, Florida. It was a great weekend. There was camping tubing and of course lots of food. My initiation that weekend was a series of pranks beginning with the shaving cream on my face. I woke up after slapping my face to swat a bug. "Thanks guys", I said sarcastically. The pranks continued all weekend.

The most memorable was the water sports. Every time I tried tubing or skiing, the boat seemed to take off so quickly, I wrecked every time. Mistake, uh no. Every time I got on the large tube or the skis I wiped out. The one of my fraternity brothers were constantly rescuing me. It was yet another part of the initiation. No seizures this time.

The end of the weekend was the welcoming of the new member to which we all received a frat shirt with our nick names on the back. Mine was "grunt". I believe that was because I was tasked with most of the manual labor and jobs no one else wanted to do. So what, I didn't care. I was happy to have some great friend who always stood by me.

I studied architecture for three years before deciding to take a break from school. Math was the reason for taking a break. I didn't think I could handle the required math to complete the degree. It was a lame excuse for not continuing on. Looking back I wish I would have completed the architecture degree.

Chapter 3-

TWENTIES AND THIRTIES

THE WEIGHT OF IT ALL

Right about the time I was taking a break from school, I had started working full time and taking my health more serious. I was working for the Broward County Clerk's Office in Fort Lauderdale, Florida.

My dad worked across the river, a short walk over the bridge. He also worked for the county government. I still didn't have my driver's license at age 25, so we rode to and from work every day. I hadn't been without seizures long enough to drive alone.

Not being able to drive was a bummer, but, in hindsight, I had one on one time to just talk with dad. We talked about work and life a lot. We decided to do something about our weight issues.

We signed up for a weight loss program and a gym membership. I was still living at home and able to keep each other accountable for our weight loss goals. We had our weekly meals and workout schedules running like clockwork. By the end of a year my dad and I had lost 180lbs between us.

We were in such great shape and feelings great about our aerobic fitness. I had maintained great seizure control and was going to be driving soon.

WORKING THROUGH IT

While I was still working at the court house, I had a seizure at work about 10am on a Tuesday. I was brought to the break room to sit down by one of my supervisors and he gave me some water to drink. Michael had asked me what happened. I told him that since I was losing weight my medication needed to be adjusted since the dosage wasn't suppressing to the seizures.

To my surprise, Michael told me he was epileptic too. He also referred me to the neurologist he went to. I used Dr. H Murray Todd for twenty three years. It was comforting to be able to talk to someone who knew how I felt. He told me about his grand mal seizures and how he fell when he was playing basketball and was knocked unconscious during one of his seizures. I told him about mine and that during mine I just look like am "on drugs" that I just stare off with a blank look on my face.

Michael said he had seen seizures like that before. I gathered that's how he knew what to do when I had one that day.

NEW REGIMENT

My new neurologist was quick to change my medications to current and more widely used anti-seizure drugs. The new meds worked great for ten plus years with only a few tweaks increasing one medication and adding another to balance the success each drug had on me and controlling the seizures. The new regiment was working great. I was on the maximum dose for Tegretol, but it was doing the job. I was taking my new medication, on time, twice a day.

One day, I remembered making the mistake of taking two doses after realizing I missed my morning dose. That was definitely the wrong thing to do. I started getting this "drunken" feeling and my sight and visual focus was that of a "vertical hold" experience. I was not stable and had to lie down.

When I followed up with Dr. Todd, my neurologist, he said, "When that occurs, go ahead and sleep off the affects of the overdose of medication". That worked just fine.

My doctor advised me that the medicine is prescribed at its maximum so doubling up is always going to have that affect.

As I continued to visit Dr. Todd regularly twice a year, He said that after my yearly blood test the medicine levels were not level throughout the day. He suggested that I break up the dosage to include a midday dose because the length of time the medicine worked was short and needed to be able to work all day. I tried the midday dose, but couldn't remember to take it. We then went back to the morning and night dosages with some adjustment to each dose. I had switched to more in the morning than at night.

I continued with my scheduled visits which were really comprised of the "balance" check. It was like I was taking the DUI test. You know hands up, touch finger to nose, turn palms up, walk a straight line and squeeze the Doctors finger to assess my grip. This was usually the first thing in the visit.

We often spoke about stressors in my life and how that was affecting my seizure control. I discovered while I was functioning at a certain level of stress over a consistent period of time, I was doing fine. It was when the stress had subsided or reduced that the seizures would occur. It seemed that my body was saying finally, I can release this tension.

LOVE LIFE?

I really wasn't even thinking about romance at this point in my life, but there was this one coworker. After repeated attempts to woo her, she said she knew someone she could introduce me to. I told her to set it up. I was looking forward to meeting her friend.

I met Kristine on a Sunday in September at a Pizza Hut in Plantation, Florida. I was so nervous. I thought she was beautiful as soon as we met. I was unusually shy that day. We stayed and ate lunch and exchanged phone numbers. It was an instant connection.

We started seeing each other on a regular basis. Our first date was to see the movie, "Ghost". We both loved it. After about two months of talking on the phone late at night and going out together, I asked her to move in with me and she said YES without hesitation.

TIME TO SETTLE DOWN

We lived together for another two months when I proposed to her in front of one of my favorite restaurants, VITA's Italian Restaurant. It was such a great place to eat. I had worked there for a few years before as a cook, so I was like family. Right before our dinner that night Kris had told me she was going to her grandmother's house in Tennessee for Christmas.

I wanted to propose before the holiday. So before dinner I said," I have to go home to get presents for my parents." What I was really going to get was the ring. I had not planned on proposing that soon in December. I was scrambling to think of what to say how the proposal was going to be answered.

She said YES! We both were so excited, that we went into the restaurant for dinner and gave the good news to my parents. What a surprise that was. They were speechless. Kris and I couldn't contain our excitement so we went dancing all night.

IT'S HAPPENING

I knew she was my soul mate. Once we committed to our life together we met with the pastor and joined the pre-marriage courses to see how serious and how compatible were as a couple. We were told to complete a questionnaire and met with a marriage counselor separately. The counselor was pleasantly surprised how compatible we were based on our meetings and questionnaire responses. We ended up deciding on a wedding date in June 1991, June 29, 1991 to be exact. The wedding was planned in about a month! Yes a month! We had met in September 1990, engaged in December and married in June of 1991. That was ten months. It was a great and fast courtship. We were both so in love with each other and were confident it was forever. In 2014 we celebrated twenty-three happy years together!!

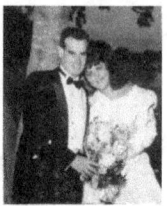

WHO AM I, REALLY?

I admit Kris didn't know everything about my epilepsy before we got married. I was still trying to hide the seizures as much as I could. Yes she should have known what she was in for! The medication was something she already knew. The seizures themselves were the mystery. Since I hadn't seen them myself, all I could teller was what I knew. I told her about loss of consciousness, the blank stare look and the lethargic feeling afterwards.

The first seizure, I was sitting in the passenger seat while Kris was driving. During that first seizure in front of Kris, I was grabbing for things around me like, the steering wheel and stick shift. Needless to say, she was really freaked out, scared and upset. She had to pull the car over to calm down and find out what had just happened. She asked me what happened and I denied it being a seizure. This was the first of many denials when seizures occurred.

After awhile, she became more and more accustomed to what my seizures looked like, when they might occur and movements I made before and after each seizure. She became more aware of them than anyone else.

STILL IN DENIAL

I could no longer deny the existence of the seizures. I knew I had them so denial was more like a statement that they weren't going to affect me in any way. She knew better. Yet, I continued the denials. She would ask, "John, are you okay?", "Are you having a seizure?" I would reply, "No!" I would try to make hand movements to distract my body from the seizure by rubbing them on my legs. I thought that it was working to ward off a seizure. I was wrong; the hand movements quickly became part of my seizures.

She was so good at spotting them that she prevented me from hurting myself on sharp objects or breaking a glass. She was always quick to remove objects from my reach. She was my angel! I don't know how she did it.

Not knowing what I looked like during a seizure made it easier for me to deny and have no remorse for the fact that they occurred at all. I had thrown up a wall before and after each seizure thinking, being unemotional about them would help me control them. It didn't work.

Kris was always right there to figure out what was bothering me or happening in my life to trigger the seizure and try to remove me from stressful situations. She wasn't always able to do that so she enlisted anyone seeing them on a regular basis to be her reporters. She, of course had the advocacy of my parents and friends. She proved her love even more by contacting my coworkers to keep an eye on me. I was quite successful. She could count on my coworkers to let her know if something was not quite right.

A NEW FOCUS

About eight years later, in my fourth year of marriage my dad approached me with a proposition. We talked about how continuing my education would pay off and further my career. He said that if I went back to school, that he would pay for the books and tuition. I couldn't resist.

Two months after school had started I broke my knee cap. I had to be in a straight leg cast. It didn't get in the way of returning to college! No way, a cast is not stopping me. I was going despite being unable to drive again.

I went to the night classes with my book bag on crutches to every class! It was interesting getting in and out of the back seats of cars. This time I was going to complete my undergraduate studies. This time the career focus was different.

I had worked as a detention cadet in the beginning of my married life. Although, I didn't continue in that role, the criminal justice system had me intrigued. I started my studies in criminal justice the fall semester weeks after my dad made the proposal about going back to college.

MATH AGAIN

As, I was reviewing the requirements of the new major of study, I realized, there it was again, math. It was the math I was so afraid of before.

I started with an advanced algebra class, the subject that I thought was too daunting years earlier. I studied like never before. I got an A! This class was the first of classes in which I was excelling in. I took every math course up to calculus and was scoring great grades in all of them.

At the same time I was taking all the criminal justice courses required by the degree and extra law classes too. It was great. I was getting an A in ninety percent of all my course work! Those I didn't get A in I scored no less than a B.

I completed my AA degree in criminal justice studies carrying two classes a semester at night while working full time.

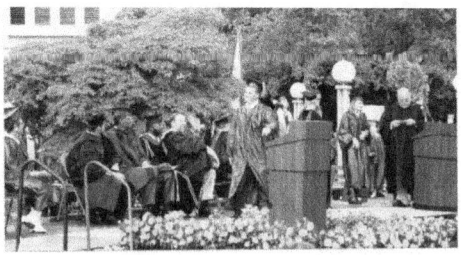

I continued from the community college to Florida Atlantic University to complete the undergraduate degree. I kept the studies going, taking the same class load and doubling up during summer to finish by the end of 2001.

DECISIONS, DECISIONS, DECISIONS

As much as I knew was bad and good for me physically and mentally, I still exercised poor judgment. In the early 'nineties my wife Kris and I had joined a civic organization to connect with some people our age. We made lots of friends. I did, however, engaged in the bad habit of social drinking. Not a good thing to mix with my anti-seizure medications.

It began as drinking at social events only. Even though, I was drinking only at party events, I regularly over did it. Most times getting sick and ruining a good time. I never moved into consistent habitual drinking but when I did it was just as bad.

The incident that ended that bad habit was a few years after starting to drink. I had gone to a restaurant on Fort Lauderdale beach. I was meeting some friends from work. They had already started drinking. The only right decision I made that night was to tell Kris to drop me off at the restaurant so I wouldn't drive knowing that drinking was going to be involved.

Once I got there, appetizers were already on the table and my friends were a number of drinks ahead of me. I stupidly thought, "I can just catch up" Catch up I did. I got so drunk that I couldn't even walk straight. I had gone to the bathroom and was still there when I was about to do a face plant into Mexican tile. My friend told me later that if he hadn't been there in the bathroom to grab my arm that the fall to the floor would have been MUCH worse. Since I did make it to the floor rather quickly, I had hit my face above the eye brow. That wasn't the only thing.

The paramedics came and Kris and my friend got me to the hospital. I of course was getting sick everywhere. Once at the hospital I had several stitches above my eye and had to have my stomach pumped. I was told by my friends and wife that my blood alcohol ratio was three times the legal limit. Stupid Stupid Stupid!!!! I could have died.

The next day I, of course, had a massive headache and hangover. I was waiting for getting ripped by my wife. The ripping never came. The waiting for it to come was worse that getting ripped. I definitely deserved it! After hearing of the night I had and the trouble I caused, that was the end of any alcohol. NO MORE EVER!!! To this day I haven't had any alcohol. Those few years of drinking were over!

Chapter 4-

THE ROLLER COASTER AND LIFE CHANGING EVENTS

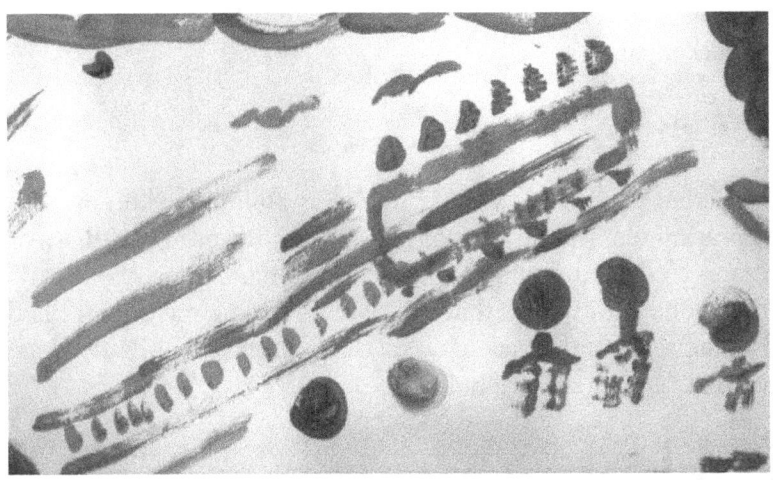

MEDICATION FAILURE

The few years that followed were filled with social events and outings regularly since we didn't have kids during the first fifteen years of marriage. It was fun. Yes there were some financial struggles but we were still young and a little reckless. The seizures were at a minimum until 2006.

I was having bad luck with cars. I had a few car accidents due to car malfunctions, misjudging distance and the sodium depletion as a side effect from one of my medications. I was coming home from work and about to make the turn down my street.

Next thing I knew, I was on the other side of the street. I had passed out. I had crossed one lane of traffic going the same direction, a large concrete median and three lanes of where oncoming traffic. This was at rush hour in the afternoon and the road was a major thoroughfare.

Amazingly by the grace of GOD, I didn't hit one oncoming car, no one was hurt and I didn't have a scratch. The only damage was to a parked car.

THE BIG ONE

Later that year, I was with family at an Italian restaurant celebrating that month birthdays. Out of nowhere I had the worst seizures to date, a grand mal. The first thing, I remember was fighting the paramedics that I felt were holding me down. I had upset the table and shocked some of my family that had never seen that type of seizure before.

My wife, daughters who were too young to remember, my parents, grandma, brother, sister and sister in law, niece and nephew were among that group. My parents, brother and sister were the only family members that had seen a seizure like this. The paramedics took me to the nearest hospital to have me examined by the ER doctors. The seizure had passed by the time we arrived at the hospital. At that point I wasn't considered a trauma patient so we waited and waited in the ER for about twelve hours. They ran tests but weren't going to admit me to stay. My wife and mother spoke up and pushed for me to be admitted over night for further testing. I was released less than 24 hours and told to follow up with my neurologist.

I did see my doctor within the next few days. We decided based on his recommendation that the meds needed to be changed and that the long time medication was not cutting it anymore.

It was also decided that I don't drive for two years which in Florida was the state law for being seizure free. I went on the new meds and started driving again two years later. At that point all was fine. That is until the move!

THE NORTH CAROLINA EXPERIENCE

My life had been a relatively normal roller coaster ride until my family and I had moved to Charlotte North Carolina in Mid 2011. The move started out to be a new adventure in our life. The ride has had bigger highs and lows than I had ever expected.

This roller coaster was the high adventure kind that makes a sharp turn after a deep plunge and you feel like you are going to fall out of the car. Seems fun for a while then when you are just getting used to the jostling the car climbs up into a loop upside down, not just once, but, several times throughout the ride.

It started off with a job that I was excited about starting as the next logical step in my crime analysis career.

It was great at first; I quickly learned that there wasn't any learning curve in private industry. With no formal training, it felt as if I had a "fire hose" had been turned on me. The influx of information about the company, the job itself and culture was overwhelming. Over the next six months to a year after arriving in Charlotte, with no close family and friends, I felt stress like never before. I began thinking what a mistake this move was.

THE JOB

I was becoming someone I didn't like. I was always stressed and paranoid about my work performance, new colleagues, new bosses and the constant demands of being "on call". It was a job function I was unprepared for and felt I couldn't ever get the constantly changing job requirements perfect. I just wanted to go back to Florida. I felt this job is hopeless; I can't meet anyone's expectations. Yes the job became so stressful and was some place I didn't want to be.

The stress brought my epileptic seizures to a level like never before, setting off a weird chain of events from the beginning of 2012. In the beginning of the year, the job goals and division operations of the job I started in June. 2011 had done a complete 180. My position became so isolated and hard to navigate the company focus and mission. It was a lonely job.

I really missed the camaraderie I had been accustomed to for the major part of my working life. I wasn't prepared for the beginning of this new wave of change in my life.

I hadn't ever seen that much change in such a short period of time in forty-four years of life, twenty years of marriage, four of those years being a father. Yes, the four years of being a father prior to moving to Charlotte, incorporated a lot of change. I was navigating the waters as you would think any fairly new parent could include the late nights. My wife and I thought, "We got this! If we could handle parenting we could handle anything." We couldn't have been more wrong!

HOW DID I GET HERE?

The seizures became more frequent and severe than ever before. I thought a medication change would do the trick. Ok, so my new neurologist, Dr. Steven Putman and I made some changes. He added another anti convulsant and something for anxiety.

We thought at first it was working, but then in August of 2012, I had a weird catatonic seizure. My wife immediately called my Dr. Putman and was in to see him the next day. My wife called my boss and she said, "Tell him to take as much time as he needs". She was the type of boss that you didn't hear from unless there was an issue of some kind.

The beginning of August 2012, Dr. Putman had some tests run, like an EEG, an MRI, and take home seizure monitor that tracked my brain seizure activity while I slept. This was the beginning of a long series of tests.

It was discovered I had scar tissue on my brain along with my increased seizure activity. I was diagnosed as having mesial temporal sclerosis as a result of years of seizures.

WHAT'S GOING ON?

I was quickly referred to another specialist the next day. The Epileptologist, Dr. Rajdeep Singh scheduled me for several tests in September.

I had MRI, SPECT, PET scans and another of many EEGs. They all came back with results of abnormalities. The EEGs were like having some weird electrically charged wig. This "wig" felt like getting used to new hair that was hot glued on.

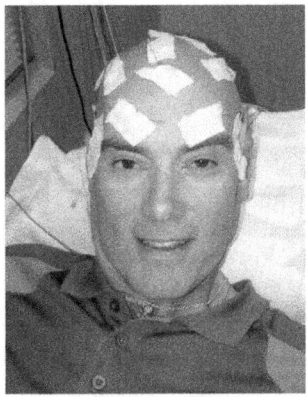

At one point I got to wear one home to sleep in. My daughters thought it was so cool that I had an electric wig.

MY FRIEND AND THE EEG

The EEGs were so regular that I had the same medical staff adhering and removing the electrodes each time. John, the EEG technician, and I were glad to see on another each time. We joked with each other about the tests and at one point we're taking pictures. I was scheduled for one on Halloween day. I was missing a work party where we all were going to dress up. I told my colleagues that I would send pictures. I had dressed up in my Miami Dolphin fan clothes. I had John take pictures of me in the EEG electrodes. I sent them to my colleagues at work to pass around the office. The pictures were a hit. There were pictures posted around the office when I returned the next day. It was great fun dressing up and the electrodes were a bonus to the costume. I was now the rouge football player.

KEEPING TRACK

I started keeping a journal of my seizures to keep the doctors apprised of the activity. I found a great epilepsy journaling app so that I could keep track wherever I happen to be. I hadn't ever kept a journal of any kind so the app made it easy. The app let me not only track the actual seizure, date and time, it gave me a chance to record how I felt physically and emotionally. It gave me a chance to really acknowledge how I had felt during and after each seizure and how my feelings about the seizures were affecting how I acted and reacted to life.

I quickly realized how the stress of the job affected my emotional well being. I couldn't believe how many partial seizures I was having on a daily and weekly basis. I was discovering how stress was really affecting my everyday life. It was great therapy and a new learning experience. I learned a lot about myself. What I really wanted work to be like and how I was coping with life.

THE SLEEP OVER

By mid November I was in for a week stay in the hospital for seizure monitoring in the ICU of the Epilepsy Unit. It was surprising to hear that all the steps needed to finding a solution usually takes six months to a year to reach the seizure monitoring. At this point, I had reached that point in three months.

During the week of monitoring in the hospital I was hooked up to electronic leads on my brain 24 hours a day and live feed video. When I arrived for check in, I felt as if I was staying at a hotel for a week. One of the first things that were done was the medicine I had relied upon every day for roughly forty years was taken away. I knew it was going to happen and gave the medicine up willingly. I was also told that every other night I was going to be sleep deprived to cause the seizures quicker.

The sleep deprivation schedule was changed to occur less because Dr. Singh said I was having too many episodes. I was also put back on some medication to enable some control of inducing the seizures. So as you can imagine, I endured the regular wake up, to have my vital signs checked.

THE STROBE

The most interesting part of the daily routine was the seizure inducing exercise. The nurse would bring in the strobe light and breathing apparatus so they could have me watch a series of strobe flashing cycles and graded breathing exercises. I had this type of test before and knew how to anticipate the strobes. I knew that the cycles were repetitive and quicker each cycle and that they were ten seconds apart. I thought I was clever for picking up on that from the first one.

The breathing exercise run at the same time as the strobe light wasn't so easy. The pattern was obvious but the performance not so. I didn't really have the knowledge for proper breathing. I was struggling with the constant increase in breathing speed and rate at which I was to continue it. So the two simultaneously run exercises usually did the trick and that was to cause an episode the staff could track.

The staff of nurses was great in accommodating my family and me to the point of bringing in an extra bed for my wife and my dad who took turns sleeping at the hospital with me.

CATCHING A SEIZURE

My wife and dad were told it would be a good idea to stay so they could help document my seizure activity. My dad was there one of the days I had a seizure that needed to be tested. This seizure was the first of many that had to be documented by a brain scan. The scans had to be taken after an injection of blue dye to capture the seizure activity. On the first occasion, I fought the nursing staff during my seizure and spilled the dye that needed to be injected in my arm to record and image of the seizure cause. That opportunity for a CT scan was lost. That didn't stop my seizures. I soon had another one.

The third day of the stay I had three seizures. During the trips to the lab for the brain scans I had another seizure on the way back to the room. Of course my vitals were constantly checked in the middle of the night and I didn't sleep well. At this point, I was thinking, "will this ever end?" I was so exhausted. I was seeing my doctors, Dr. Singh and Dr. Waataja daily.

The last day in the ICU unit I asked to see a video of one of my seizures from the hospital stay. Yes, a weird request. I hadn't ever seen what my family and friends had seen multiple times. Dr. Singh thought it was an unusual request too. I told him I wanted to know what my family had to endure during my seizures. After I viewed the video, I was surprised that the seizures weren't more obvious to others. It was a great relief to know and see what my seizures actually looked like. They were not as severe as I had created in my mind.

HOORAY, SURGERY

This is where the roller coaster makes the turn that you just can't wait for. It's like looking for the light at the end of the tunnel for some relief and that light being at the end of the corridor around that turn you were looking for.

I finally realized that all of the tests were leading up to brain surgery. Then I had an A-Ha moment, oh brain surgery maybe the solution.

During all of the testing and hospital stay, our new church was constantly praying for God's grace. It was to the point that we had people praying for seizures to happen during the week in the hospital of seizure monitoring. They would look at us with the "you want us to pray for seizures? Well if that's what you want, then we will pray. This round of testing and all the ones that followed through January 2013 became hoops of fire to jump through. Each test was another step closer to brain surgery.

The church was there the whole way. I was really touched and amazed at the pastors and prayers from Forest Hill Church. I was visited by fellow Christians from my church almost daily while I was in the hospital for monitoring WOW!! I couldn't believe the support! Brain surgery became the end goal. Yes it was being cheered for by my family and more by me!

WHAT TO DO NEXT

I even had a WADA test where each side of my brain was put to sleep one side at a time. It was a "little bit" of a strange feeling being awake only on one side at a time. Creepy and scary at the same time but the doctors were there at either side of me during the test. Most people would be freaking out at all these tests. I, on the other hand was welcoming these tests. Yes, I was excited at the prospect of having brain surgery. I did all the research and watched all he videos of the surgery, still with open arms.

THE SURGERY OPTIONS DISCUSSION

The time came to find out if all the tests were going to conclusively be decided by a board of surgeons that I was an absolute candidate for the surgery. It was like waiting on pins and needles to find out the board's decision. The neurological board recommended that I undergo the surgery.

I was told during the consultation with my Epileptologist, Dr. Singh, that my brain had "rewired itself" to function around the seizure activity. Now that's self preservation! He also told me that I had a choice to make. He said, "You can have a surgery that enables electrodes to be put on the brain tissue to locate any additional areas that may affect memory, motor skills or any chance of possible side effects of the surgery and a second surgery to remove the affected area of the brain." "Or" he said you can have just the surgery to remove what we know is the affected area." I said, "wait a second, aren't you the doctor?" "Why are you asking me?" He said "I have to ask for your permission to do either surgeries or just one". "It is because even though the surgery is needed, it is still considered voluntary". I said, "What's the difference if I have one or two surgeries?" He said, "Having two surgeries provides for further mapping of the brain which will give us more specific details". "But, of course two surgeries have a higher risk of infection from foreign objects touching your brain and the surgery itself." I said, is it possible to have the same results from just one surgery?"

He said, "The surgical board of neurologists is confident where the problem area is and the one surgery should have the same result we are looking for." I immediately told Dr. Singh that since you are sure of the problem area, I see no reason not to just go with just one surgery. He said, "Since you are electing the one surgery, I am ordering additional surgical mapping during that same surgery to get the best possible results." "The neurological board and I agree on the course of action and main concern and risk is long term memory loss possibility, but we are confident that it will not be affected."

SCHEDULING THE SURGERY

It is now mid January 2013, in the office of the neurosurgeon, Dr Michael Heafner, that was going to perform the surgery. He was of course, informing me of all the potential risks and possible benefits of the surgery. That day I found out the actual name of the procedure. The clinical name was right temporal craniotomy for anterior temporal lobectomy and amygdalohippocampectomy. The research I did described this surgery as possibly two separate surgeries. Even if I hadn't done the research, I was still confident that this was the best route. I agreed without hesitation to have the surgery and as soon as possible! It was to be on February 20, 2013 at noon.

Once the date was set, my excitement increased. Finally I was going to have the possibility of being free of the "cage" the seizures had kept my brain in. The hope this surgery was leading me to be thankful of the experiences good and bad that helped me to this stage in my life. I had been praying that the light would appear.

My family was hopeful and worried at the same time. My wife, Kris who is my biggest supporter was great at getting everyone praying about all the consultations, tests and the surgery.

You would think I would be a nervous wreck; no not me I couldn't wait for the day to come to get on with what I believed was going to be a new life.

THE DAY HAS COME

It was surgery day! I was up and ready for "high noon"! My parents had been in town a few days and were at the hospital with my wife. My church had been amazing there praying at every service, visiting me in the hospital and even bringing meals to my family and me.

This day was to be a great day! We arrived at the hospital and checked in about ten thirty am. We were told to go to the waiting area. I sat with my Dad, my Mom, wife Kris, and my church pastor awaiting the call to be prepared for surgery. Finally, my number was called to get ready for surgery. The first stage was being taken to have the surgery prep started. The hospital staff did the usual prep, vital signs, restatement of the surgery process and understanding.

For the first time in my life, I was drawn on my head with a sharpie. I said what is that for? My Neurosurgeon, Dr. Michael Heafner said it was for the actual incision points. The marks were shaped like big question mark on my head.

As, I was wheeled in for surgery, I took a moment and said to GOD, "I trust you got this, I am not afraid. The results will be as you intended." I was just in a great place, knowing that HE was in control. I wasn't nervous at all!

Once I was in the operating room, I asked, "I am getting a discount right?" "My head is already shaved." The surgical staff was quite surprised at my optimistic outlook about the success of the surgery I was about to undergo.

THE WAITING

The surgery took about four hours from first cut to last suture. I was in the recovery room for about two hours when I saw my wife. I stayed in the hospital for another day in ICU for observation and then to my surprise was released to go home. The surgeon told me that they removed a golf ball size piece of my brain on the right side. I thought well now I have room for more brain growth.

The scar I had after the surgery was a bit hideous.

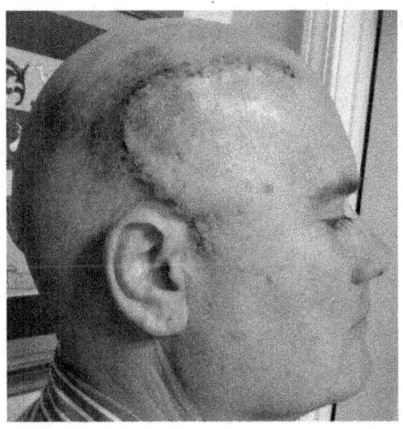

THE RECOVERY

The next few days following the surgery were the hardest. I couldn't open my jaw since the surgery required my jaw muscles to be cut. I had such a wicked headache that it seemed no amount of medicine would help! I remember that I felt like I needed to get my own drink and food. I didn't do that often since I slept most of the time and when I did get something to eat it was something small since my appetite hadn't returned yet.

My parents stayed in town until my birthday which was the second time they had come to stay with us since September 2012. I had made it known that day that now I had another milestone like my birthday for which I was now forty-six.

It was like a rebirth and the start of the new me. The surgery resulted in a new and improved brain. So I was born and reborn on an odd year. Go figure, I am a little "odd" anyway. I now had this large scar on the right side of my head from the top around to the front of my ear in the shape of a question mark. I thought cool I am the "riddler"!

My meals for the first month or so were Greek yogurt and anything that I could eat that wouldn't require me to open my jaw too wide or chew. I was doing a lot of laying around which drove me crazy. I needed to do something.

Chapter 5-

RACE FOR LIFE

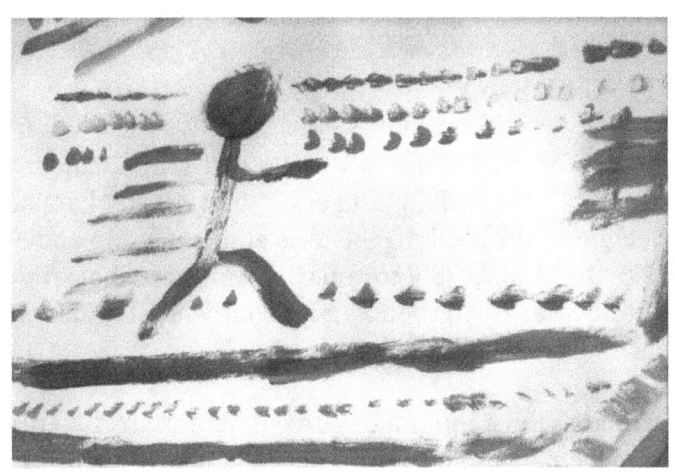

THE COMEBACK KID

My wife had started a new job. We were a one car family and the girls needed to get to the bus stop every day after my wife had to be at work. I met the same group of moms there each day. I joked about being the house husband. They were a great and supportive group. At first I was walking them to the bus stop not far from the house in our hilly complex with a cane. You know the kind that could have had tennis balls on the bottom. That only lasted about a month when I said. "You know what, I don't need this cane"!

About the same time my eldest daughter, Meghan said, "Why are you fat, daddy?" Well, I didn't see that coming! I was caught off guard and thought that was mean to say. I replied back to her, "good question". It was then that I decided I had enough of this being fat stuff. I am going to have to do something, but what!

I had been walking without the cane for a week or so of when I had a great idea, I was going to walk and get my coffee! Mind you, the place for coffee was about a mile and a half away.

GETTING SKINNY

The group of moms thought I was crazy. I said, "Time to get rid of this weight". "I'm walking to get it. So every day I walked to get coffee after I dropped off the girls at the bus stop and every day said to the moms, "Got to walk!" I walked to the coffee shop got my coffee, sat down for about an hour while I drank my coffee and walked another mile and a half back home.

I was walking three miles a day five days a week. I then started walking to the park, stores restaurants and many other places, most of which was two to three miles away. That brought my walking up to about 20 miles a week.

I also started major portion control, yogurt and banana in the morning and sliced meat or tuna at lunch.

In the beginning, I cut out the bread and soda. The soda hasn't returned to my diet to this day. Walking and dietary changes jump started my weight loss.

By mid April, just two months after surgery, I had lost twenty pounds! I then decided to up the mileage.

ANTE UP

For the next two months I increased the weekly mileage about five miles and sped up the pace. I started back at work in mid June which was great! I didn't realize that until I started going to work that I have would have to change my workout times. I was taking the train to work every day and there were several stops in the area where I got off to walk to the office. The walking helped but it wasn't nearly as much mileage that I had been covering. I thought that I would just walk to stops further from the office to get some more walking in. This was not working as I expected.

So I decided that I would have to walk after work. I started each night about two hours after I got home. During the two hours, I was of course dedicated to meet the family needs like my girls' dinner and homework. The good news was that with all the walking I was gradually losing the weight I wanted to get rid of.

By the time I vacationed in Florida in August 2013, where I had lived for Forty-four years of my life prior to moving to North Carolina. I had gone from 247lbs to 177lbs. A whopping 70lbs loss!

HITTING THE MARK

I had reached the goal of seventy pounds I set to reach by the Florida trip. I had a little more incentive from the bet I made with my eldest daughter, Meghan, that I could do it. It was great to hear how great I looked. I had found my ego which I thought was lost.

I had returned to the weight I had when my father and I dieted together and lost 180lbs between us. While on vacation, my dad and I walked in the evening to get some more mileage and take advantage of having quality time with my dad alone to talk.

Oh, I forgot to mention, the whole time I was walking I had been wearing knee braces to protect my right knee. I hadn't exercised my knee that much since my car accident in 1995.

JUST CHECKING

For the next year and a half after the surgery, there were several post surgery follow up appointments. I saw my neurosurgeon, Dr. Michael Heafner twice after the surgery. I saw him for the one week follow up and a month later for the suture removal. I was wondering during the sutures removal was in going to have a scar. I really thought it would be cool to keep my question mark shaped scar. A permanent reminder of the amazing things my brain had done before the surgery and the things it will do from now on. I really wasn't going to mind if it was extremely obvious. I was happy with what it signifies.

I also had the pleasure of seeing Dr. Singh, Dr. Johnnie Waataja and staff three more times since the surgery, every six months. The first follow up in early September of 2013 was to check how recovery was going. The doctors reduced my medicines by one medicine that visit.

The second visit, at the one year anniversary mark the doctors were surprised by the weight loss and improved fitness that I had attained since the previous visit.

PUSHING HARDER

When I returned home I continued to walk the same routes and increasing the mileage to eight miles at a time in about one and a half hours. I was happy about my stamina and endurance and felt great! After a few nights of the six, seven and eight mile walks, I thought there has to be something else.

Still using my braces, I wonder what running would be like. On September 3, 2013, I started running for the first time in my life! I started with a mile a few times and was worn out.

I then started pushing harder working up to two mile runs and trying to beat my time each time I ran. It was working. I was still spent at the end though. This went on for about two weeks, when I decided to run farther. It became three mile runs away from the house and walk back.

I was still wearing the braces and couldn't stop running and start again because if I took a break I was done running for the day. Realizing this I started running farther before I stopped for the day. By the end of September I was running four miles at a pretty steady pace, about 37 minutes.

I found myself obsessively researching everything about running from form, pace, speed and distance. My tablet had so many websites save on my home screen I was constantly moving around and compressing them into folders to make room for more. In October, I started my five mile runs to about 51 minutes and lengthened my runs to six and seven miles in a little over an hour. By this time the weather was getting significantly colder, into the 20's, 30's.

A RACE YOU SAY

Dr. Johnnie Waataja couldn't believe it. She said, "Wow you are amazing! You lost seventy pounds and started running?" I said "yeah I ran four miles last night." She said, "you know there is a 5k for Epilepsy on November 2nd". I said, "Cool! I'm there!" A couple of days before the 5K my total medicine dosages were to be cut in half over the period of two weeks.

On my way to being medicine free! The most recent and third follow up visit was great, again! I was told by Dr. Singh that the cause of all the seizures and epilepsy was from two cells that didn't develop correctly before birth. So that means these two "rouge cells" as I am referring to them, are the cause, not the fall from the crib.

Dr. Singh said, "We can reduce the medication. Which one do you want to cut?" "Wow, I get to decide? I thought for sure one of the ones you are having me chose from was going to be the last one to go." I said excitedly. He said, "It doesn't matter which one of the two. The last one to be cut is telling one we haven't adjusted yet.

THE SLIDE

So I chose another of my three medications and the dosage for it was cut in half. Wahoo! I was seeing the second chance to start over without losing my past memories and have another major milestone to share becoming a reality! I saw a chance to leave behind the scared and self conscious person I once was. People were saying, that's inspiring, amazing, that's great news. I couldn't believe the comments and words of encouragement from people I didn't even know. The complements always came as a surprise. All I could say was thank you. They meant so much more. I was having a hard time believing that I was amazing or inspiring.

RACING ANYONE?

On November 2nd, I ran my first 5k for Epilepsy and finished it in 28 minutes, and was fourth one to finish.

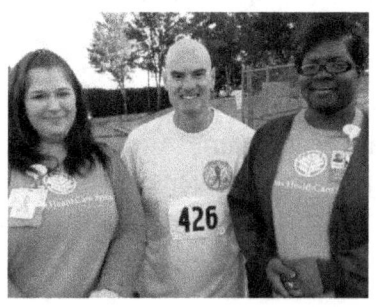

I have to admit most of the participants weren't there to race. I saw some of the staff that attended to me while I was in the hospital for a week being monitored for my seizures. It was great to see them there and they couldn't believe how thin I was. My wife was the one who recognized them before me. By my next race on Thanksgiving, I had lengthened my long runs to eight miles in an hour and twenty one minutes.

IT'S ALL IN THE TIMING

On Thanksgiving Day, I ran my first timed race for a distance of four miles in South Charlotte North Carolina, an area called Ballantyne. I had done my best four mile time that day. It was my first official timed race. I finished in 37 minutes and 40 seconds, recording my first personal record (PR).

My in laws were in town for Thanksgiving that week; my brother in law had made a surprise visit that week. On the day of the Turkey Dash race my father and brother in law came to the race. They were amazed that I had become a runner and that I finished in the middle of the pack of about 800 runners.

I was so thrilled, I had dropped my per minute mile to 9:29 from 10:48 in two and a half months. I had so much to eat that day. I felt so good about my running achievements at this point that I was trying to recruit anyone that wanted or seemed interested. I was so excited to run every day. I am sure that my talking about running became annoying to my coworkers. Still I couldn't help myself. I was even sharing my half marathon and marathon goals.

RUNNERS EVERYWHERE

By the end of the year, I had really started to notice all the runners in the Charlotte, North Carolina. So much that I was seeing them everywhere on any day of the week. My daughters started counting them while we were out and about. My wife said, "Look what you started". "Not me, they started it" I said. Ok, so maybe, I prompted it most times.

I had made another visit to Florida for Christmas and had a great time with my family for a week. My family had said they were so proud of my achievements. My brother had said, "you wouldn't catch me doing three miles". I was so surprised to hear him admit it. I always thought he was the one who enjoyed sports and being outside more than me. It finally dawned on me that I enjoy it too now!

That week I had told my family that I had decided about a month earlier that I was going to run a half marathon on March 9, 2014. The last week in December 2013, my dad and I went out early in the morning while everyone else as still asleep. The day before and after Christmas about seven am I ran and my dad trikked, which was a quasi bike/roller blade that involved moving forward using a side to side turning styled motion called "carving". He would trikke and I would run.

GETTING LOST

It was the first time I had run in the heat and humidity of Florida which I had grown up in. It was hard and frustrating to run. The first few times I ran during the holiday week I had actually run a faster pace than I had been running in Charlotte, N.C. I was amazed and proud of how I could still keep improving on my time. I did my longest run to date on December 27 2013 of nine miles in 01:33:58.

During that week of Christmas, it was kind of fun exploring a new running route. The day of the nine mile run I had made a turn that did not follow the route that my dad and I had mapped out the day before. I hadn't realized that I turned too early until I was well off course. My dad told me he had tried to follow me but was blocked. I had turned into a housing development with security at the gate. My dad had called me on my phone and asked if I knew where I was. I told him no, but, I would find my way.

I had gone so off track it took me over a mile away from our planned course. I had run far enough around until I found the main road. I called my dad and suggested he meet me along the road towards the house. I saw where he had parked to meet me, looked at my distance ran and waved him on to catch me further down. I wanted to squeeze in an extra mile.

FLORIDA WORKOUTS

It was great getting up each morning earlier than anyone else in the house to exercise like we would years earlier. I didn't realize how much I had missed the workouts with my dad. After I came home I ran my first ten mile run on January 1, 2014 in fourteen degree weather in a time of 01:33:51. Wow, my first ten mile run and I ran a mile longer and faster than my nine mile run by seven seconds. It was such a good day to run! It was cold but fun, even when I ended the run and was walking to cool down it was really a cold walk since my core temperature wasn't as warm. In other words walking two miles back to the house I was FREEZING my butt off, but it was so worth it. I repeated a ten mile three more times but couldn't beat or duplicate the time. It was really frustrating.

I wanted to be able to finish the half marathon in two hours. I thought maybe.

THE RACE

The half marathon was two months away. I didn't get in as many runs as I would have liked since Charlotte had such bad weather, like it hadn't seen in ten years. It was snowing for a few days closing the schools and pretty much the whole city.

It was the first time for my daughters to see snow! It was awesome playing in the snow with them. I had been fit since August of the 2013 and was thankful that I was able to run and play with them and some neighbors out front, throwing snowballs and making snowmen. My wife and I hadn't seen snow in quite a while ourselves so it was equally fun for us as well.

During February and the first week of March I had a lot less runs than previous months and was getting worried that I was going to lose the endurance I had built up. I was still obsessing about a finishing time but all the research and runners I spoke with said "don't worry, just finishing was an accomplishment". I agreed but my ego was still saying come on you can do it in two hours despite what all of the pace calculators were telling me.

The night before the race, I went with my family to the Charlotte Motor Speedway to pick up my shirt and bib number. I was excited because the race as early the next day.

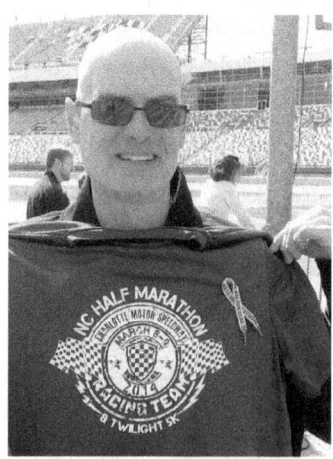

START YOUR ENGINES!

The day of the race, I was so excited that the night before I couldn't sleep and was up before my dad who was an early riser anyway. My parents had driven all the way from Florida a few days before, on my birthday, to see me race. I wasn't even sure what my plan was for food consumption to get ready for the race was going to be. I ended up eating my usual morning routine of yogurt and banana. I figured I needed more than that so I ate an energy packet and a bagel.

I was ready to go with my running clothes and my racing number pinned to my shirt that I had set out the night before. I wanted to be there early but too early for the rest of the family so my dad and I went on ahead to the Charlotte Motor Speedway where the half marathon was taking place. Surprisingly, I wasn't nervous at all.

When we got to the track, we set up a good place for my family to see me race. I went into team waiting area and walked with the other runners to line up for the start at 7:30am. I spoke to some of the other racers about where they were from and how much they had raced before. For some, it was their first time and others were seasoned racers. Still, I didn't think I was nervous.

REVING UP

I kept telling myself to start slow so I wouldn't burn out halfway through the race. I started off almost toward the back of the racers thinking I didn't want to be passed often because I was too slow.

I didn't realize until after the race that I could have started closer to the starting line. I started off slowly as I had consistently practiced. It felt as if it was too slow. I felt good through the first half at the six mile mark which the racing timers mark your pace for the first half of the race.

I felt fine and was running based on how I felt and wasn't obsessing about my pace. I was getting Gatorade at every water station and didn't eat any mid run food that I had packed in my belt for just the occasion. I didn't think I needed it. I wasn't fatigued at all.

So far in the race, I hadn't taken any walk breaks. It was straight running. I had passed a few runners that I knew had gone out before me at the start. That felt so good that I knew I wasn't going to be in the back of the pack.

I kept looking for the leaders and was slowly increasing my speed after the halfway mark to try to catch up. At mile marker eight my dad and youngest daughter had positioned themselves to see team runners as they went by. They had just moved close enough to the fence to see me go by. I gave my daughter a wink and thumbs up as I saw them and the signs they had made to cheer me on for the race.

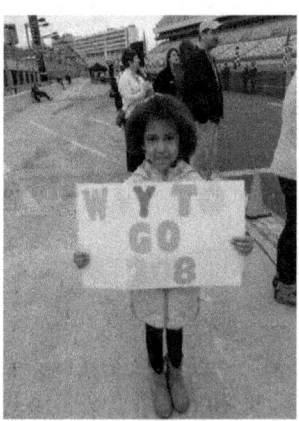

HITTING THE GAS

I felt more refreshed after seeing them. It was only at mile 10 that I actually slowed down for a few seconds to walk. I told myself, "no walking" and quickly resumed my pace.

Around mile marker eleven I heard some racers talking to each other about "finishing strong" and took that as a challenge to speed it up more towards the end. I was running at a good pace for me.

I remember looking at my watch and thinking, "there goes my target goal"," ten minutes until the two hour goal finish time and I have two more miles to go". I remember thinking "would have been nice to get this goal", "so let's see how close I can get"! I cranked up my speed about that time. I was pushing as hard as I could.

I sprinted the last half a mile to the finish line. As I crossed the line I saw the number 02:17:06 as I went under the marquee. Wahoo!!! I crossed the finish line thinking, "THAT WAS AMAZING"!!!! Why didn't I start running earlier in life? I was so hungry and thirsty and was glad I stopped for Gatorade at every station. I met my parents, wife and daughters near the recovery tent and grabbed many bagels and bananas to eat. They asked how I was doing. I said, "AWESOME"!!! "Let's go again, one more time around!".

They gave me that, are you crazy look! I said, "yes really let's go!" I felt a feeling of euphoria, which I have never felt before. I went to see how I placed on the time rankings anxious to see how I did. The time I saw was my finish time from the "gun" starting the race. I finished better than two and a half hours!!!!

I got my racing medal. It was so cool. It was a race car with spinners and blinking lights.

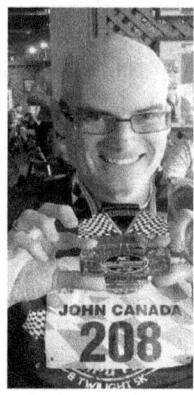

I also discovered in the race times that I finished the second half of the race faster than the first!! To top off the ego pumping, I found that my finish time based on the chip timer attached to my race number, that my finish time was 02:15:37 (two hours, fifteen minutes and thirty-seven seconds)!!!!!

Could it get any better?!?! I was thrilled and so incredibly proud finishing my first half marathon. What a great accomplishment!!

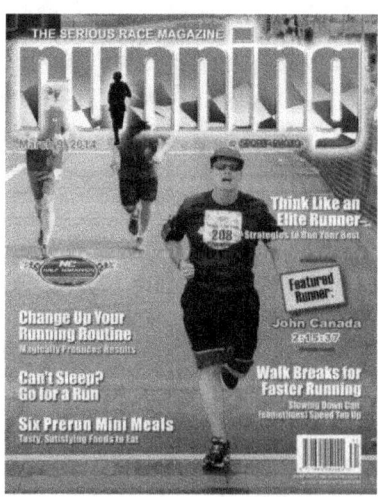

Chapter 6-

NEW LIFE

NOT EXPECTED

The race was a culmination of efforts. I would have told you I couldn't do it if you would have predicted this a year earlier. I was not really one who shared my experiences on social media, but that day I was posting statements like, "Race fans, I am happy to report the results of the race are...." I could believe the amount of supportive comments from my friends that some of which I hadn't spoken to in a few years. Some comments from my closer friends were, "you are a runner, now? Awesome", "Run John run!!", and on and on they went. My ego pumping continued for the next month or so. I even purchased a photo from the race promoters. I picked the one showing me stepping on the finish line with my finish time with the background being the cover of a racing magazine! I couldn't wait to scan it, email it, post it and text it to my friends. My family thought wow he is on a magazine.

My brother in law even responded to the email I sent with, "is this real"? I responded back with, "IT IS TO ME!!!"

BUCKET LIST

I got so excited about having personal goals to look forward to that I started a "bucket list". What's on the list you say? Well here you go. 1. Half marathon. 2. Marathon. It looks like I can knock off one and two by the end of the year.

In 2014, I had completed a half marathon in March and had registered to run a marathon in November. 3. Hot air balloon ride.

4. Windsurfing. 5. White water rafting. North Carolina has a renowned center for it. 6. Skiing. 7. Hang Gliding. 8. Hiking. This was most likely the next on the list. 9. Surfing. I always wanted to try surfing but was too afraid of "wiping out". Not anymore. I say bring it on. 10. Scuba diving. Another I was afraid of because of my epilepsy.

Yeah, pretty crazy right? Why not? If I can handle everything else in my life so far then I could handle this event. What it's an hour of my life? What's the worst that could happen?

I have faith that whatever God's plan for my life. His plan is going to be as it is intended to be no matter what. These days anything could be possible.

WHAT NOW?

I was thinking about the November marathon. At first, I thought 26.2 (miles) is double what I just finished. Wow could I really do that?!

I was still thinking about the next event when I spoke to a mom that was picking her kids up at school he same time I was. We started talking because I noticed she was wearing a shirt from a previous race she had run. I told her about my first half marathon and that I had registered for a full marathon. She thought it was great that I finished the last 7 miles faster than the first than the first six. She said, "That's not easy to do. That's a great achievement for your first distance race"! She said, "You should do the full marathon! Your body will remember the endurance of the half and that it can be done. Make sure you build up your long runs to twenty miles and you will be fine". That conversation gave me the confidence I needed.

I will finish a marathon by the end of 2014! I seem to find a lot of runners in Charlotte North Carolina. They are willing to have a long conversation just because they overheard me talking about running. It seems to be a magnet for starting conversation and advice. Speaking of advice, running has been great for networking for personal and professional growth. Just joining a running social media group has paid off. I'm getting all kinds of great suggestions on how to train. Of course, training is not without its own set of challenges, like running in the heat of summer, the steep hills and the even longer weekly runs.

ADJUSTING

Amidst all the constant changes my wife and two daughters are so tuned into my running schedule that they are always asking me, "Are you running today?"

Adjusting my running locations and times since our move was getting more and more interesting and finding new routes in a new city and joining my first running group since I started running. It's a great group of people to run with, share experiences with and enjoy the run. They also keep me motivated, focused on my marathon training and goals and keep me accountable.

Training in this new location is nice with the rural, family and homey feel to it. The hills are more rolling, steeper elevation and not as many sidewalks.

Day time running becomes the new schedule. It does have the great benefit of more tree coverage and ability to run in the roads since the traffic is less busy than my previous neighborhood.

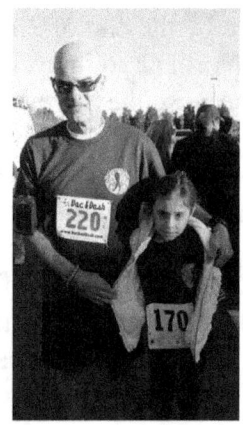

A DAUGHTER'S ENTHUSIASM

While my daughters were in Florida for the summer my mom had mentioned that I was going to run marathon in November. Meghan, my eldest daughter said," I want to run 26.2 with you, dad!" I told her if you want to we have to practice. We can start with a 5k first. She agreed.

So the first Saturday after she came back from vacationing in Florida with their grandparents Meghan and I went for a half mile run/walk. I let her lead the training that day. I didn't want to be discouraged and think that it was too hard. I wanted her to run because she wanted to. So far she seems to like it a lot!

She had heard about the club at school called Girls on the Run and wanted to do it. I was so glad that she wanted to do something like her dad!!

We are training for a 5k in November 2014 and she joined Girls on the Run, a program for youths interested in running for sport and fun.

She found the form and details the first day of school. She wanted to have all the clothes for running. I told her she needed running shoes and comfortable clothes.

She was looking in all the stores for the clothes and shoes she needed to wear. I am so proud of her commitment to do something she seems genuinely interested in.

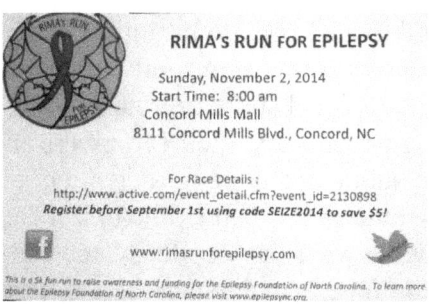

RIMA'S RUN FOR EPILEPSY

Sunday, November 2, 2014
Start Time: 8:00 am
Concord Mills Mall
8111 Concord Mills Blvd., Concord, NC

For Race Details :
http://www.active.com/event_detail.cfm?event_id=2130898
Register before September 1st using code SEIZE2014 to save $5!

www.rimasrunforepilepsy.com

This is a 5k fun run to raise awareness and funding for the Epilepsy Foundation of North Carolina. To learn more about the Epilepsy Foundation of North Carolina, please visit www.epilepsync.org.

GETTING THE WORD OUT

I ran in the 5K race last year called Rima's Run for Epilepsy. Rima and her daughter are both affected by epilepsy. Rima and I shared a common bond. I was amazed that she decided to organize the race instead of having a birthday party. She wanted to give back.

She had told me she was overwhelmed by the request by runners asking if she was holding the race again next year. She decided to continue the race for a second year. She was excited that the race was being held in a better location which was going to get more exposure for Epilepsy Awareness.

I told her I wanted to be a part of it. We met regularly and discussed how I could help support her. She gave me flyers and sponsor sheets which I passed out the flyers to local runners, running groups and businesses to sponsor the race.

Rima had all the sponsors from the previous year return for the 2014 run. This year's run included timing for the runners. This was a great accomplishment that Rima and I had worked on. The race was a huge success. The runner turnout was over double from the previous year. All the proceeds from the race went directly to the Epilepsy Foundation both years to benefit patient care.

I feel like I need to give back to promote Epilepsy Awareness. I will continue to look for the opportunity to get involved with the Epilepsy Foundation, local support groups, being involved in events supporting patients and their caregivers and bringing awareness to the public about the needed attention for support. I really believe that the gift of being able to run has helped me to embrace that I will always have epilepsy and can make a difference and continue to understand how everyone is affected differently.

I consider myself fortunate enough to be a voice for others. Epilepsy most of the time is misunderstood and can go unnoticed by the public. Epilepsy is a very real condition in which some have multiple seizures on a daily basis. Not enough people are aware of epilepsy and I hope to change that one person at a time.

FOR LIFE

You know what; I haven't been this passionate about sports or personal goals in a while. I rediscovered the competitive spirit I forgot I had. I don't ever want to stop running for racing or personal recreation. This is a sign of how running will play a big part in who I am now and where I am going personally and professionally. The running location for racing or training no longer matters.

The sport is so addictive that I will adapt to any environment be it weather or surface conditions. No matter what the day brings I have a "runner's high" most times I finish a run. I am still in awe that running gives me a boost every day. It raises my mood and confidence in my abilities.

I am still constantly researching running as much as I scan for professional advice on form and training. So far in has been what you would call "self taught". I am very pleased how that has worked for me! I am always on the hunt for races.

I found a great race on the beaches of North Carolina for the marathon in November 2014 one week after the Epilepsy run. I also plan on running in another half marathon in January 2015. Yes, it's a lot of racing. I love it!!! So racing to the next personal record I go! So race fans stay tuned for the next race results!!!

Chapter 7-

THE BIGGEST CHALLENGE

THE MARATHON

The day had come to put all of my training into one long run. I had been training for this chance to take on another running challenge. I signed up in early October 2014 to run a marathon in the Outer Banks of North Carolina. This course was across the cities of Kitty Hawk the home of the Wright Brothers first flight, Kill Devil Hills and Manteo, North Carolina.

The course was going to be a challenge because I had to run two and a half miles of trail, and a high bridge. It was scheduled for Sunday, November 9, 2014. At mile ten I would be entering Hags Head Nature Preserve for two and a half miles of trail running. Crossing the 85 foot tall and 1 mile long Washington-Baum Bridge would be the last of two challenges in this marathon.

PRE-MARATHON

I left Waxhaw, North Carolina on Saturday, November 8th to head to the Outer Banks. It was a 6 hour drive with my wife, daughters and parents in tow. We left early enough to get to Kitty Hawk around 4pm. It was just in time to pick up my bib number, racing shirt and the entire packet goodie bag items.

When I arrived at the expo for the Outer Banks Marathon, I noticed so many runners and families walking around talking to the vendors. There were so many new accessories that could improve my running experience. I noticed the bib numbers 0 through 50 were reserved for the elite runners. It was exciting to get my race number which made the race real. There was no turning back now.

DON'T OVER THINK IT

When I arrived at the starting line at 6:45 am, ready to run my first marathon, I was overwhelmed by the number of runners at the starting line. My dad and my eldest daughter, Meghan went with me to the starting line to watch me head out. We walked around a little to see the different runners and groups ready to getting ready run. When it was 7:10 am, I said see you later to my dad and kissed my daughter.

At 7:20am the gun was fired to start the race. The elite runners started off as the rest of the runners edged up to the starting line. I started off towards the back of the pack to keep my self from starting off too quickly. I had trained my self to begin my pace slowly. I started running slow enough to feel like an easy run. The sky was overcast and it was about fifty degrees, perfect for running. I even decided to forego wearing a hat since it seemed as the sun wouldn't be out that day.

SETTING THE PACE

I looked ahead at the groups of running packs; each had a pacing runner with a sign of an expected finish time. Initially, I was training for a finish time between 4:45:00 and 5:00:00. My target time was to complete the run by noon which would have been 4:20:00. Yes, a bit ambitious. It seemed achievable at the time. I started off slowly as planned and then I spied the pacer with the 4:30 finish time. I was talking to another runner who was talking about returning to his previous finish time. I asked him why and he said he was much younger then. We kept pace for a mile or two when I decided to catch up with the 4:30 pacer group. The pace felt great and I kept with the group through mile 10. My form felt great and I was on my way to reaching my goal. At mile 8 we all ran past the Wright Brothers Memorial in Kitty Hawk. This was the second city in the race behind Kill Devil Hills.

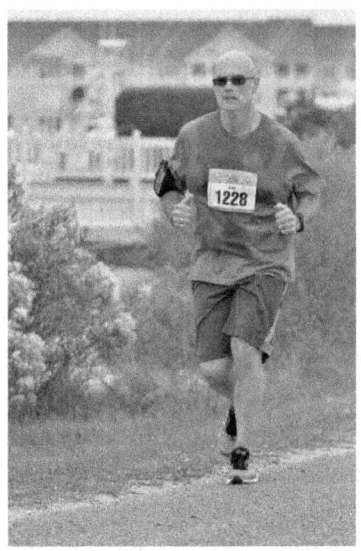

THE TRAIL

The first challenge I encountered was the trail portion of the race. I had read that is was a packed dirt trail. I thought, "I can do this, it shouldn't be too bad". I did not train much for trail running. Once I reached the beginning of the trail, it seemed more rocky and loose than expected. I noticed a lot of runners were slowing down and walking. The trail became narrow quickly. Well now seems as good as any to take a walk break and stay with the group. The tree cover and woods were nice and cool and a nice change of scenery. I was thinking to myself, "This trail seems longer and hillier than I pictured". At mile 12, I ramped up my effort and came out clear of the trail at mile thirteen.

My half marathon time was 2:20:26.5 which was longer than my half marathon race in March. It wasn't where I wanted my half marathon split to be. It's a marathon, the goal today is to finish.

SECOND HALF

It's time to start the second half of the race. Now that I was back to road running the course felt easier. The trail definitely took a toll on me. The trail being behind me, I was more optimistic about the second half of the race. As we all wound back out to the main course the 4:30 pace group was getting away from me. I was feeling disappointed that my goal time was slipping away. I was able to keep telling myself that this was my first marathon only 14 months after beginning to run and 8 months after my first half. I decided to reset my goal back to finishing the race. It was going to be a personal record no matter what. I ran solid until mile 18 before I took a walk break. The weather continued to remain perfect for a marathon. I quickly picked up the pace again so that I wouldn't "hit the "Wall". I believe I escaped the feeling of exhaustion at mile twenty. I was actually feeling euphoric. I am still running and can make it to the end. At, that point I was unable to see any more pace group signs. I didn't really pay attention to my watch. I just kept moving.

POWER BUTTON

The support from the people along the course continued to be amazing. Just knowing that I was getting support from people I didn't know cheering me on was awesome. I saw this one family who had made a sign that said "Power Button" and had a big red circle in the middle of the very large poster board. I ran past the family who was cheering on the runners as they past the sign. Each runner tapped the poster board to get a boost.

When I got near I tapped the button too. I tapped a bit too hard though. I had knocked the poster board out of the little boy's hand. I stopped to return the poster board to the boy. I felt I needed to give it back for the other runners to use as a boost. The family cordially said, "Don't worry about the sign just keep running".

That made me feel better that I could have just kept running without any hard feelings about knocking the sign away. I was just focused on finishing the race at that point and was determined to continue enjoying the run. It was the furthest I have ever run and it felt great.

THE BRIDGE

As I arrived at mile 22, I saw the second challenge. It was the Washington Daub Bridge which spanned across the Roanoke Sound. It seemed like a huge mountain to climb. I had trained for big hills and suspected I could climb this one too. It was a staggering 85 feet high at its crest with a steady grade. Ok so it was bigger than I had trained for. I had underestimated the seemingly flat course challenges. I wasn't going to be defeated though. I kept on climbing the bridge at a steady pace keeping up with the group that was around me. I had chosen one runner in specific to stay close pace with. We continually passed each other until the finish line. I was a great game to play to keep me motivated. At mile 24, I had made it to the third city in the race, Manteo. Upon passing the sign "Welcome to Manteo" I knew the finish line was within reach. Two miles away was the finish line through the city. As I got closer to the finish line I could hear the cheers of the runners and supporters as they crossed the line. The last mile was great. I could see the finish line around the last block.

MY SUPPORT TEAM

As I got closer the runners were thinning out. When, I was about 50 yards away from finishing the race. I was greeted by my daughters Meghan, who had run her first 5k a week earlier, and my younger daughter, Brianna, the sprinter. They were both calling me. I asked what they were doing not realizing that my wife, Kris had sent them to meet and finish with me. Brianna said,

" Just want to hold your arm to the finish, daddy". Meghan said, "I will beat you to the end". At that point, I was in sprint mode to finish strong. I said to my girls, Ok, let's go. I was able to finish with my girls. It was unexpected and awesome.

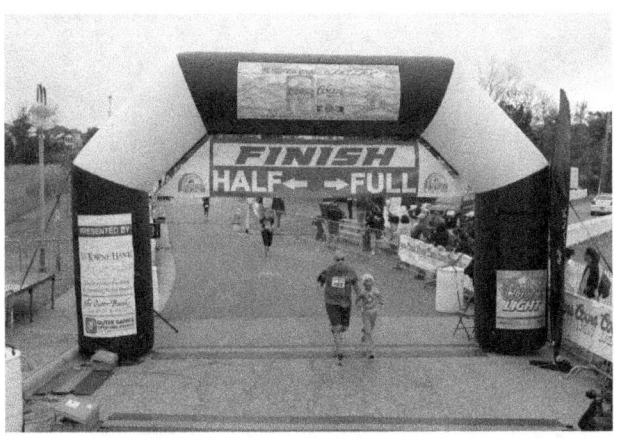

HOW DID I DO

After I went through the finish line I grabbed my finisher medal, water and a few bananas. As I walked around, I felt like I was walking on a cloud. I had finished in 5:26:05. It wasn't my goal time but so what I finished. To my surprise, in the second half of the marathon my last three miles were the fastest. My training had paid off.

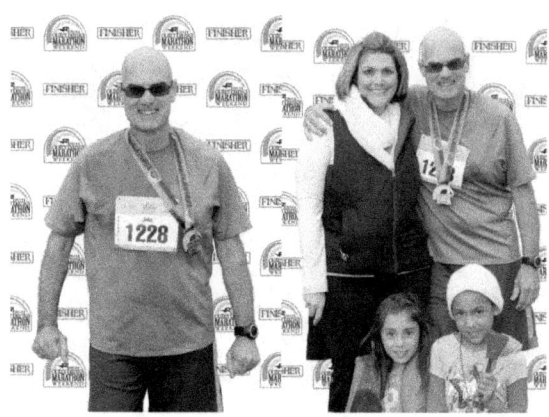

I was now a member of a very small group of Americans who even attempt this feat. Only 1% of Americans would even attempt to walk, let alone run a marathon. I couldn't have ended my first full year of races without the training and support of my family. This has been a great year in 2014 to prove that I could be seizure free, maintain my new body, and run some long distances. The new year of 2015 will bring many new racing goals and challenges. If I could accomplish my distance goals of 2014, I can reach any goal I set my mind and body to accomplish.

MAKING A DIFFERENCE

A few weeks after the marathon, I had relocated back to my home state of Florida. I hadn't been home two weeks when I was contacted by Claire Hosmann, on December 1, 2014. She is the

Clinical Public Relations Representative for Carolinas Health System. She emailed me about being interviewed by FOX46 which is the Charlotte affiliate for FOX News. She also said that the Carolina Health Network wanted to interview me as well.

I was quite taken back and excited at the same time. "OMG I am going to be on TV in Charlotte." Claire even mentioned that the interviews would include videos of me running.

Claire and I were emailing back for a few days to determine if the interviews could be set up the same day. We had confirmed FOX 46 interview would take place at 10 am on December 5th 2014 in the Epilepsy Monitoring Unit of the Charlotte Medical Center Main Hospital. The Carolina Health Network interview was in the same place at 1pm the same day.

Everything was set except getting to the interviews. I was in Florida and needed to be in Charlotte four days later. I was so excited that the drive to Charlotte, North Carolina from Fort Lauderdale, Florida, which takes 12 hours, didn't faze me.

The day before the interviews my Dad and I took turns driving to Charlotte. We arrived at Pastor Robbie Fischer's house to stay the night. Pastor Robbie had been a great support for my family while I was going through the events leading up to the surgery.

The morning of the interviews, I was surprisingly relaxed. I was excited to be seeing Dr. Singh again after just a few weeks. My Dad and I arrived at the hospital where I had my surgery and grabbed a cup of coffee in the café on the first floor.

We were waiting in the lobby for Claire to meet us when she texted me. I jokingly said to my Dad, "She is probably right behind me and I don't know it." She was. We waited for Caroline

Fountain, the reporter from FOX 46. She greeted us and the four of us took the elevator to the monitoring unit on the ninth floor.

When we got there we were greeted by the Epilepsy Monitoring Unit (EMU) staff. Just a few minutes later, Dr. Singh met with us and proceeded to an empty hospital room. We all gathered in the room awaiting the beginning of the interview.

Dr. Singh was interviewed first for a few minutes. During the joint interview, Dr. Singh and I were discussing my upcoming 2 year anniversary on February 20 2015. I will be seizure free for two years. In our discussions, Dr. Singh said that if I had been seizure free for two years after surgery it was unlikely that I would have another seizure. I thought not having another seizure would ever be possible.

I was interviewed next. I wasn't nervous at all. Caroline was a great reporter. I felt at ease just telling her about myself, living with epilepsy, brain surgery and my passion of running. It didn't even feel like I was even being filmed.

After the interview, Caroline Fountain took me outside to film me running for the interview. It was forty-four degrees out and I was just wearing running shorts and shirt. Everyone else was bundled up. We went to the breezeway and Caroline filmed some running.

The first interview was completed at 11:30 am and I felt elated. Caroline told me the interview would air that same night on FOX News Charlotte at 6pm and 11pm.

http://www.myfoxcarolinas.com/story/27560099/overcoming-epilepsy-to-become-marathon-runner

We took a break for lunch and waited for the second interview at 1pm. My Dad and I talked about how the interview went. My Dad, Claire Hosmann and Caroline Fountain stated that I had done a good job interviewing.

At 1pm sharp Claire Hosmann, my Dad and I had returned to the EMU for the second interview. We were greeted by the Carolina Health Network team. Natalie McIver interviewed me to showcase a success story of the Carolina Health System doctors and staff. Dr. Singh and I were both interviewed again. This time, the video is set to be aired on Carolina Network News February 2015.

After the interview, I returned to the breezeway for some final running video. Natalie, my Dad and I chatted for a few minutes. We thanked each other for the opportunity to interview and be interviewed. Dad and I said our goodbyes and started our 12 hour trip back to Fort Lauderdale.

On our 12 hour trip home my Dad and I talked a lot about my opportunity to make a difference for Epilepsy awareness. I discovered how much Epilepsy goes unnoticed. November every year is designated Epilepsy Awareness Month and purple is the color. One in twenty-six people are affected by Epilepsy in their lifetime.

Being affected by this neurological disorder myself, I had decided that I needed to be more involved in the cause. I started by getting involved with the local races supporting epilepsy. I had come up with the idea of organizing a distance race for the Epilepsy Foundation of Florida and starting a blog about epilepsy and running.

THE END

ABOUT THE AUTHOR

John is a native born Floridian with a beautiful wife and two amazing daughters. He has a passion for epilepsy awareness and a new found love of running. He went to college at Florida Atlantic University, earned a bachelor's degree in criminal justice. He lives his life through his faith in GOD and belief in himself. He encourages others in their accomplishments whenever he can. He participates in social media in groups that challenge his goals of running and epilepsy advocacy. He enjoys spending time with his wife, daughters and parents. John likes to work his brain often with puzzles and games; he is a bit of a math geek. He has come to realize that life is precious and every moment matters. He believes, "if you cannot see the light at the end of the tunnel, change direction or turn the corner. You may just find the light in an unexpected way".

www.ingramcontent.com/pod-product-compliance
Lightning Source LLC
Chambersburg PA
CBHW070606290526
45790CB00002B/805